UNDERSTANDING

FUNCTIONAL

MEDICINE

Unlocking Optimal Health: A Comprehensive Guide To Transform Your Health Vitality, Explore Key Concepts, Targeted Approaches, Targeted Strategies And More

DR. KARSON BRYAN

DISCLAIMER

This book's content is meant to be used solely for general informative purposes. Despite having taken every precaution to guarantee the content's accuracy, the author disclaims all duty and responsibility for any errors or omissions. It is recommended that readers exercise caution and, if needed, seek expert guidance. Any and all liability for losses, damages, or other outcomes arising from the use of the material included in this book is disclaimed by the author and publisher. All referenced product names and trademarks are the property of their respective owners and are merely cited for identification. Any likeness to real people or things is entirely accidental. Since it is a work of fiction, this book should not be used as a substitute for professional, legal, or medical advice. It is advised that readers seek advice on particular issues from qualified experts."

Please make sure that this disclaimer is modified to fit the particular requirements and subject matter of your book. Seeking advice from a legal expert is also a smart option if you have any questions or require a more thorough disclaimer for your specific book.

TABLE OF CONTENTS

CHAPTER ONE

FUNCTIONAL MEDICINE

INTRODUCTION

Functional medicine is a comprehensive approach to healthcare that prioritizes understanding illness and disease's underlying causes over treating its symptoms. This marks a significant turning point in the medical sector since it provides a thorough and patient-focused approach to treatment. The ideas of Understanding Functional Medicine, The Principles of Functional Medicine, The Evolution of Functional Medicine, and How Functional Medicine Differs from Conventional Medicine will all be covered in this introduction.

KNOWLEDGE OF FUNCTIONAL MEDICINE

Instead of focusing only on treating symptoms, functional medicine is a patient-centered, systems-oriented approach to healthcare that aims to find and treat the underlying causes of disease. It acknowledges that every person is different and that a variety of complex interactions, such as those involving genetics, lifestyle, environment, and mental health, affect an individual's health. By reestablishing equilibrium and enhancing the body's inherent processes, this method enables the body to mend and stay healthy. In-depth examinations and extensive diagnostic testing are frequently used to identify the precise imbalances or dysfunctions that exist within a person's body.

THE FUNDAMENTALS OF HOLISTIC HEALTH

Multiple fundamental principles form the basis of functional medicine. The idea that the body has the innate capacity to repair itself under the correct circumstances is one of the core beliefs. Additionally, it emphasizes the need for a relationship between the patient and the healthcare professional, in which the latter works closely with the former to develop a customized treatment plan. Rather than only treating symptoms, functional medicine aims to address the fundamental causes of disease. It also acknowledges the interdependence of the body's systems, realizing that a malfunction in one might have repercussions that are felt widely throughout the entire body. It also encourages the emphasis on lifestyle issues and prevention as vital aspects of healthcare.

THE DEVELOPMENT OF HOLISTIC HEALTHCARE

Over the past few decades, functional medicine has developed in reaction to the drawbacks and shortcomings of the traditional medical paradigm. Although its roots are in the 1960s, it became a separate field in the 1990s. Several variables, including the rising realization of the shortcomings of symptom-based methods, improvements in medical research, and the growing significance of tailored care, have contributed to the development of Functional Medicine. The area is always evolving, incorporating new scientific discoveries, technological advancements, and therapeutic approaches to keep up with the ever-changing healthcare environment.

HOW CONVENTIONAL MEDICINE AND FUNCTIONAL MEDICINE DIFFER

The way that functional medicine approaches healthcare is very different from that of conventional medicine. A disease-centered model is frequently used in conventional medicine, with an emphasis on treating particular diseases or their symptoms. Functional medicine, on the other hand, adopts a patient-centered strategy, attending to each person's particular requirements and circumstances. Functional medicine emphasizes dietary adjustments, lifestyle modifications, and natural interventions to assist the body's healing processes, while traditional medicine typically uses pharmaceutical medicines and surgery as the main treatment techniques. Additionally, it uses cutting-edge diagnostic testing which is less frequent in conventional medicine to find underlying imbalances and dysfunction.

Functional medicine is a cutting-edge approach to healthcare that places a strong emphasis on individualized, patient-centered treatment and a thorough comprehension of the underlying causes of disease. Practitioners of functional medicine seek to assist the body's natural ability to heal itself, avoid disease, and advance general wellness. It is still evolving, bringing in the most recent scientific findings and technological advancements to provide patients with all-encompassing, efficient, and holistic healthcare solutions that deviate greatly from the traditional medical paradigm.

CHAPTER TWO

THE BASIS OF INTEGRATED HEALTH

THE METHOD FOCUSED ON THE PATIENT

Functional medicine is based on the patient-centered approach, which is a key idea that distinguishes it from conventional medical procedures. Under this paradigm, the emphasis is on identifying and treating the illness's underlying causes rather than only treating its symptoms. The patient-centered approach acknowledges that every person is different, with their unique combination of lifestyle, genetic, and environmental factors influencing their health. Putting the patient at the center of their healthcare process gives them the confidence to actively participate in their health.

TURNING THE ATTENTION TO THE PATIENT

Moving past the reductionist perspective of sickness that frequently characterizes traditional medicine entails turning the focus to the patient. Functional medicine looks for the interrelated web of elements that affect a patient's health condition rather than focusing only on treating individual symptoms. This methodology recognizes the intricacy of the human anatomy and the diverse ways in which different systems and factors interact. The goal of Functional Medicine practitioners is to promote long-lasting health and vitality by exploring the deeper causes of disease.

ESTABLISHING A HEALING ALLIANCE

Developing a therapeutic alliance is a crucial component of the patient-centered methodology. Under functional medicine, the patient and the physician collaborate to identify the underlying problems that might be causing the patient's health problems. Active listening, empathy, and a thorough comprehension of the patient's goals, lifestyle, and medical history are hallmarks of this partnership. To support the patient in navigating their health journey and making knowledgeable decisions about their care, the practitioner takes on the roles of advocate, educator, and guide.

PERSONALIZED HEALTH CARE AND PATIENT SELF-DETERMINATION

The two main tenets of functional medicine are patient empowerment and personalized care. Personalization refers to adjusting interventions and therapies to each patient's particular needs and situation. This method acknowledges that due to variations in heredity, environment, and lifestyle, what suits one individual may not be appropriate for another. Functional Medicine seeks to create more lasting and effective results by using a customized strategy.

The foundation of the Functional Medicine paradigm is patient empowerment. It is encouraged for patients to take an active role in managing their health and making decisions. People are given the information, resources, and encouragement they need to make wise decisions regarding their health, such as dietary and lifestyle adjustments. Patients who feel empowered are more inclined to take charge of their health, which improves treatment compliance and results in better health.

The core ideas of Functional therapy are centered on the patient, emphasizing the patient, forming therapeutic alliances, accepting individualized therapy, and empowering patients. This paradigm encourages a more thorough and efficient approach to healthcare by acknowledging the individuality of every person and attempting to identify the underlying causes of disease.

CHAPTER THREE

MEDICINE BASED ON SYSTEMS AND ROOT CAUSES

DETERMINE THE ROOT CAUSES:

Finding underlying causes is a key idea in the field of medicine and healthcare that directs the use of systems-based medicine. It entails taking a thorough approach to diagnosing and treating medical disorders, looking below the obvious symptoms to identify the underlying reasons. Practitioners of systems-based medicine look for underlying causes of a patient's health problems and attempt to solve them rather than just treating the symptoms.

This method highlights how important it is to take into account a variety of factors, including genetics, lifestyle, and environmental influences, that may contribute to health issues. It motivates medical personnel to learn more about the patient's background, lifestyle, and habits to acknowledge the possibility that a single symptom or ailment may have several related causes. Through the identification of these underlying reasons, medical professionals can customize treatment plans for each patient, resulting in more long-lasting and efficient approaches to better health.

THE VALUE OF SYSTEMATIC THINKING

Since systems thinking are the foundation of systems-based medicine, it is an essential idea. Systems thinking acknowledge that the human body is a complex, interconnected system with numerous interdependent components, as opposed to focusing on isolating specific symptoms or illnesses. This holistic viewpoint recognizes that modifications or problems in one region of the body can impact other systems profoundly, sometimes resulting in symptoms in other parts of the body.

Healthcare practitioners are encouraged by systems thinking to see patients as dynamic, integrated wholes rather than as a collection of discrete components. It necessitates an awareness of the interactions and influences between the several components of an individual's health, such as environmental, mental, and physical aspects. By enabling practitioners to recognize the connections and interdependencies across various facets of health, this method paves the way for more efficacious treatment plans that target the underlying causes of health issues.

GENETICS'S PLACE IN FUNCTIONAL MEDICINE

Functional medicine, a branch of systems-based medicine that aims to prevent and promote health by treating the underlying genetic elements that contribute to each person's distinct health profile, heavily relies on genetics. Healthcare professionals can better grasp how a person's genetic composition can affect their reaction to certain therapies and how susceptible they are to particular diseases by studying genetics.

Healthcare practitioners can customize their therapies to better meet the individual needs of their patients by looking into their genetic predispositions. Potential health hazards can be identified with this tailored method, which also enables early intervention and the creation of risk-reduction plans. Comprehending genetics is crucial in functional medicine to deliver more accurate and customized care, potentially resulting in better health outcomes.

THE MATRIX OF FUNCTIONAL MEDICINE:

A key tool in functional medicine and systems-based medicine for thorough patient assessment and treatment is the Functional Medicine Matrix. It is a framework for organizing and assessing a patient's medical history, symptoms, and possible underlying causes. A timeline of the patient's medical history, a matrix of significant clinical imbalances, and a patient-centered assessment are some of the essential components of the matrix.

Practitioners can methodically investigate a patient's health conditions about their environment, genetics, and life experiences by utilizing the Functional Medicine Matrix. It makes it possible for medical experts to find correlations, patterns, and possible underlying causes, which promotes a more comprehensive and individualized approach to treatment. Clinicians can use this matrix as a guide to better grasp the complexities of a patient's health and create individualized treatment plans.

INTRODUCING THE FM MATRIX

Several important categories, such as antecedents, triggers, and mediators, are commonly included in the Functional Medicine

Matrix. The term "antecedents" describes the environmental, lifestyle, and genetic elements that have shaped a person's health throughout their life. Triggers, which include diseases, traumas, and stressors, are particular occurrences or circumstances that either cause or worsen health problems. The physiological and biochemical imbalances that show up as illnesses or symptoms are known as mediators.

Healthcare professionals evaluate and identify particular elements pertinent to the patient's case within each of these areas. This methodical approach guarantees that no possible underlying cause is missed and aids in the creation of an all-encompassing and customized treatment strategy.

CASE STUDIES AND THEIR USES

Examining real-world uses through case studies can help one fully appreciate the benefits of functional medicine and systems-based medicine. These real-world examples show how healthcare professionals successfully handle complex health situations by applying these concepts.

Case studies shed light on the methods used to determine underlying causes, apply systems thinking, and include genetic data. They demonstrate the customized approach provided by systems-based medicine, in which treatment regimens are made specifically for the individual needs of every patient.

Systems-based medicine provides a comprehensive and individualized approach to healthcare. It is guided by the ideas of uncovering underlying causes, systems thinking, and the integration of genetics. With this method, the Functional Medicine Matrix is a useful tool that helps medical professionals identify underlying issues and create individualized treatment plans. Healthcare professionals can enhance patient outcomes and advance long-term health and well-being by looking at case studies and putting these ideas into practice.

TOOLS FOR DIAGNOSIS AND TESTING

A key component of medical practice is comprehensive patient assessment, which entails obtaining and evaluating data to completely comprehend a patient's health status. In addition to evaluating physical symptoms, this procedure takes a comprehensive approach that takes into account psychological, social, and environmental aspects. Healthcare providers can find possible risk factors, underlying medical conditions, and lifestyle choices that may be influencing a patient's health difficulties by doing a thorough patient evaluation. Healthcare professionals can make better decisions about diagnosis, treatment, and overall patient care by carrying out a comprehensive assessment.

A vital component of the thorough patient evaluation is the analysis of the patient's medical history and lifestyle. It entails a thorough investigation into the patient's prior medical history, encompassing illnesses, surgeries, prescription drugs, and medical family history. In addition, lifestyle analysis looks at psychosocial variables including stress levels, sleep patterns, and occupation in addition to a patient's habits like food, exercise, smoking, and alcohol intake. To comprehend the patient's general health and identify relevant risk factors and lifestyle-related causes to their current health condition, this information must be gathered.

A diagnostic strategy that goes beyond conventional clinical laboratory testing is called functional laboratory testing. It is centered on evaluating the bodily functions of the patient, including immune system performance, hormone balance, nutritional condition, and metabolic functions. Functional testing offers important information about underlying dysfunctions or imbalances that conventional lab testing could miss. Hormone panels, dietary sensitivity testing, thorough stool analysis, and advanced lipid profiles are a few examples of functional tests. With the use of these tests, medical professionals can determine the underlying causes of illnesses and create more specialized treatment regimens.

The process of evaluating the information gathered from thorough patient evaluations and functional laboratory tests to reach a definitive diagnosis is known as interpretation and diagnosis. To identify the root cause of a patient's health difficulties, healthcare providers must interpret the results in light of the patient's medical history and lifestyle. Clinical knowledge and the capacity to make connections between test findings, symptoms, and the patient's overall health picture are prerequisites for this stage. When diagnosing, it's critical to rule out the possibility of several contributing causes and distinguish between primary and secondary problems.

CHAPTER FOUR

NUTRITIONAL EVALUATION

DIETARY EVALUATION AND SUGGESTIONS

An essential part of determining a person's nutritional status and general health is dietary analysis. It entails a methodical assessment of an individual's food intake to comprehend nutritional consumption, eating patterns, and possible excesses or deficiencies. This evaluation aids medical specialists in providing well-informed advice for enhancing a person's diet and general health, such as registered dietitians and nutritionists.

Usually, the first step in the dietary analysis procedure is gathering comprehensive data regarding an individual's eating habits. This includes keeping track of meal frequency, portion sizes, food and beverage types and quantities, as well as any special dietary requirements or preferences. meal diaries, self-reporting, and more sophisticated techniques like meal frequency questionnaires and 24-hour dietary recalls can all be used to collect this data.

The next step after getting this data is to evaluate the diet's nutritional value. This entails figuring out how much is consumed in terms of macronutrients (proteins, fats, and carbs) and micronutrients (vitamins and minerals), as well as assessing the diet's general quality and balance. To help with these computations, a variety of instruments and software are available, improving the accuracy and efficiency of the procedure.

Personalized dietary suggestions can be given by healthcare specialists after the completion of the dietary analysis. These suggestions might focus on addressing certain health issues or illnesses, promoting a balanced diet, optimizing nutrient intake, or correcting deficiencies. Guidelines for portion management, meal planning, food selection, and dietary adjustments based on each person's particular requirements and objectives may be included in the suggestions.

TESTING FOR MICRONUTRIENTS

Micronutrient testing is a diagnostic technique that evaluates a person's vitamin and mineral levels. Although macronutrients proteins, lipids, and carbohydrates—provide energy, micronutrients are crucial for many physiological functions as well as general health. Iron, calcium, and zinc are a few examples of minerals, as well as vitamins like C, D, and B12.

Micronutrient testing is important because imbalances or deficits in these vital nutrients can cause several different health problems. Individuals with certain dietary limitations, abnormalities of absorption, or long-term conditions that may impair the absorption of nutrients can benefit most from testing. Deficits might be detected with its assistance before they become symptoms or health issues.

A blood sample is usually required for testing, while some procedures may also require samples of urine or hair. The amount of particular vitamins and minerals that are present in the subject's body is determined by analyzing the sample that was taken. The individual's levels of these micronutrients are then compared to reference ranges that have been developed to ascertain if they are adequate or deficient.

Healthcare providers can create tailored recommendations and treatments to correct any problems found after the data are released. This could entail dietary adjustments, supplementation, or other therapeutic approaches intended to raise micronutrient levels and enhance general health.

NUTRITIONAL THERAPY IN INTEGRATIVE MEDICINE

Functional medicine is a branch of medicine that goes beyond treating symptoms to identify and treat the underlying causes of illness. Functional medicine places a great deal of emphasis on therapeutic diets, which use certain nutritional approaches to manage or prevent a range of medical diseases and improve wellness. These diets are tailored to the particular requirements of each person and frequently focus on particular areas of health.

The elimination diet is a popular therapeutic diet in functional medicine. This entails eliminating particular foods or dietary groupings that might be causing a person's health issues, like autoimmune illnesses, allergies, or sensitivities. To find out which foods cause negative reactions, these may be progressively reintroduced over time.

The low-FODMAPS diet, which is frequently used to treat irritable bowel syndrome (IBS), is another such. This diet, which is adapted to each person's tolerance levels, limits specific fermentable carbs to alleviate gastrointestinal discomfort.

CHAPTER FIVE

HORMONAL AND ENDOCRINE EVALUATION

NATURAL HORMONE BALANCING

An all-encompassing strategy for enhancing the body's endocrine system without turning to medication is natural hormone balancing. Hormones are essential chemical messengers that control metabolism, development, mood, and reproductive activities, among other physiological processes. Hormone imbalances can cause a variety of health problems, including mood changes, weight gain, exhaustion, and even chronic illnesses like polycystic ovarian syndrome or thyroid abnormalities.

Keeping a healthy lifestyle is one of the most important methods for achieving natural hormone balance. This includes getting enough sleep, exercising frequently, and maintaining a nutritious, well-balanced diet. Hormonal health can be supported by eating a diet rich in vital vitamins and minerals, such as omega-3 fatty acids, vitamin D, and B vitamins. In addition to lowering stress, physical activity can help maintain a healthy weight, which is essential for hormonal balance. Additionally, getting enough sleep is essential for the body to repair tissues and control hormone production.

Another crucial component of natural hormone balance is stress management. The endocrine system of the body can be upset by prolonged stress, which can result in abnormalities of hormones like cortisol and adrenaline. Methods like yoga, deep breathing exercises, and meditation can support hormonal balance and lessen the negative consequences of stress. Hormone homeostasis also depends on limiting exposure to environmental pollutants, such as the endocrine-disrupting substances included in some plastics and pesticides.

Supplements and herbal treatments are frequently used to naturally balance hormones. For generations, people have utilized herbs such as chasteberry, black cohosh, and maca root to treat hormonal issues, especially in women going through menopause or irregular menstruation. But before using herbal supplements, it's crucial to speak with a healthcare professional to be sure they're secure and suitable for your needs.

ANALYZING AND TESTING HORMONES

Understanding a person's hormonal status and treating abnormalities in hormones need hormone testing and analysis. These tests, which assess the levels of hormones in the blood, urine, or saliva, are usually carried out by medical specialists. The particular hormones being evaluated as well as the person's health issues will determine which testing procedure is best.

Hormone testing is most commonly done by blood tests. They offer a moment-in-time view of the bloodstream's hormone levels. Various hormones, including thyroid hormones, sex hormones (estrogen, progesterone, testosterone), and adrenal hormones (cortisol, DHEA), are evaluated based on the symptoms and concerns. These tests' results assist medical professionals in diagnosing hormonal imbalances or illnesses and customizing treatment regimens.

Tests on saliva and urine are occasionally done to evaluate particular hormones. For example, saliva testing can shed light on the patterns of hormone synthesis throughout the day, which is important information to know when it comes to disorders like adrenal fatigue. A more thorough understanding of hormonal activity can be obtained by using urine testing to obtain information on hormone metabolites.

Because hormones frequently change throughout the day and can be influenced by a variety of circumstances, interpreting the findings of hormone tests takes knowledge. A medical professional will decide whether hormone replacement therapy or other therapies are required after taking into account the patient's symptoms, medical history, and test findings.

THERAPY USING HORMONE REPLACEMENT

A medical procedure known as hormone replacement therapy (HRT) replaces or supplements the body's natural hormones to treat symptoms brought on by abnormalities in the hormone system. Although it can also be used for other hormone-related disorders, HRT is most frequently used to treat menopause-related problems in women, such as hot flashes, vaginal dryness, and mood swings.

HORMONE REPLACEMENT THERAPY COMES IN TWO MAJOR FORMS

1. Hormones that are chemically identical to those the body naturally produces are used in bioidentical hormone replacement therapy

(BHRT). Usually obtained from plant sources, these hormones are tailored to meet the unique hormonal requirements of each individual. Though research on the safety and effectiveness of BHRT is still underway, it is thought to have fewer negative effects than synthetic hormones.

2. Conventional Hormone Replacement Therapy: In conventional HRT, hormones that are not generated by the body are substituted by synthetic hormones. Although this method has been used extensively in the past, there are certain hazards involved, including a higher risk of breast cancer, stroke, and blood clots. However, in certain situations, the advantages of traditional HRT frequently exceed the disadvantages, and medical professionals carefully consider the advantages and disadvantages for each patient.

The choice to get hormone replacement therapy (HRT) should be taken after consulting with a healthcare professional because it is a very customized treatment. They will take into account things including a person's medical background, present state of health, and the intensity of their symptoms. HRT can be given in a variety of ways, depending on the individual and the particular hormones being replaced, including tablets, patches, creams, gels, and injections.

Achieving natural hormone balance necessitates taking a comprehensive strategy that includes stress reduction, lifestyle changes, and natural therapies. Hormone replacement therapy can be a useful option for treating severe hormonal imbalances; the choice of treatment method is highly personalized based on an individual's needs and health considerations. Hormone testing and analysis are crucial for understanding an individual's hormonal status.

CHAPTER SIX

STRATEGIES FOR TREATMENT

The integration of lifestyle and behavioral interventions is crucial in holistic healthcare since it tackles not only the physical but also the psychological and emotional dimensions of well-being. These treatments cover a broad spectrum of tactics intended to manage chronic diseases, encourage healthy lifestyle choices, and avoid sickness. They are based on the notion that lifestyle decisions and actions have a significant influence on general health. Lifestyle interventions frequently concentrate on topics like stress management, alcohol moderation, sleep hygiene, and quitting smoking.

Health education is one of the main components of behavioral and lifestyle interventions. Healthcare providers engage with people to increase awareness of the significance of making healthy decisions and to give them the resources and knowledge necessary to make adjustments for the better. To assist people in identifying and overcoming obstacles to forming healthy behaviors, behavioral therapies frequently incorporate motivational interviewing, cognitive-behavioral therapy, and other psychological strategies. These therapies work especially well for treating behaviorally-based chronic illnesses such as obesity, addiction, and other conditions.

NUTRITION AND DIETARY MODIFICATIONS

An individual's general health and well-being are greatly influenced by their food and nutrition choices. The body needs certain nutrients for growth, energy, and the maintenance of different body processes, which are provided by a healthy diet. Dietary adjustments can be made to achieve a variety of health objectives, such as controlling weight, treating chronic illnesses, or enhancing athletic performance.

Dietitians, nutritionists, and medical experts collaborate with patients to create individualized food regimens. To promote health and wellness, these strategies could involve modifying portion sizes, food selections, and macronutrient ratios. The significance of maintaining a balanced diet full of fruits, vegetables, whole grains, lean meats, and healthy fats is frequently emphasized in nutrition and diet adjustments. Depending on a person's needs, specific diets like the Mediterranean diet, low-carb diets, or plant-based diets may be advised.

EXERCISE AND MOVEMENT THERAPY

A healthy lifestyle must include both forms of physical activity and movement therapy. Frequent physical exercise has a substantial positive effect on mental health and general well-being in addition to assisting in the maintenance of physical fitness. Exercise can improve bone and muscular strength, increase metabolism, improve cardiovascular health, and help with weight management. It is also essential for the management and prevention of long-term illnesses like obesity, diabetes, and hypertension.

Exercise programs can be customized for each person's needs by medical professionals, physiotherapists, and personal trainers, who will consider the person's age, fitness level, and specific health objectives. Exercises for the heart, muscles, flexibility, and balance may all be a part of these programs. Exercises that involve movement therapy, like Tai Chi or yoga, can be very useful for lowering tension and increasing flexibility.

STRESS MANAGEMENT AND MIND-BODY TECHNIQUES

Keeping one's mental and emotional health requires both stress management and mind-body techniques. Numerous health problems, including digestive ailments, mental health difficulties, and cardiovascular problems, are frequently attributed to stress. Mind-body techniques integrate the mind and body to promote relaxation and lower stress levels. Effective methods for reducing stress include progressive muscle relaxation, deep breathing techniques, and mindfulness meditation.

Alternative therapies including massage therapy, chiropractic adjustments, and acupuncture are also included in mind-body practices. These therapies are intended to improve general well-being and ease physical suffering. These methods aim to establish a harmonic balance between the mind and body by acknowledging their connection. Their efficacy in addressing ailments such as persistent pain, anxiety, and depression has been demonstrated, endorsing a comprehensive medical strategy that considers the mental and physical facets of well-being.

CHAPTER SEVEN

HERBAL MEDICINE AND NUTRACEUTICALS

NUTRITIONAL SUPPLEMENTS IN FUNCTIONAL MEDICINE

Functional medicine is a branch of medicine that aims to treat the underlying causes of illness rather than only its symptoms. In functional medicine, dietary supplements are essential since they can promote many facets of health and well-being. These supplements are frequently used to support certain health objectives, close nutritional gaps, and enhance general wellness. In functional medicine, the idea behind dietary supplements is to maximize the body's functioning through the use of vitamins, minerals, herbs, and other natural components.

To address nutritional deficiencies that may be a contributing factor to chronic illnesses or imbalances in the body, practitioners of functional medicine frequently suggest dietary supplements. For instance, those who are vitamin D deficient may be offered supplements to improve their mood, immune system, and bone health. It's frequently stated that omega-3 fatty acids, which are frequently included in fish oil supplements, can improve cognitive performance, lower inflammation, and support heart health.

APPLICATIONS OF HERBAL REMEDIES

Using the therapeutic qualities of plants, botanical medicine incorporates herbal remedies as a fundamental component. These treatments are well known for their wide range of uses and have been utilized for centuries in many cultures. Plants are used in herbal therapy to treat a variety of illnesses in different forms, including teas, tinctures, capsules, and salves.

Since herbal treatments frequently address several facets of well-being, their holistic approach to health has made them especially well-liked. For example, ginseng is prized for its adaptogenic effects on stress and energy levels, while chamomile is recognized for its relaxing and digesting qualities. Turmeric is a popular choice for pain and inflammation management because of its anti-inflammatory qualities, and Echinacea is frequently used to enhance the immune system.

DOSAGE AND SAFETY CONSIDERATIONS

It's important to take dosage and safety into account when using herbal medicines and nutritional supplements in a functional medicine setting. The danger of side effects is reduced and therapeutic effectiveness is ensured with the right dosage. This is particularly crucial because taking too many vitamins or herbs could have unexpected negative health effects.

Dosage recommendations are frequently influenced by variables including weight, age, sex, and the particular medical condition being treated. Practitioners of functional medicine adopt a customized approach, customizing dosages of supplements and herbs to meet each patient's specific requirements. Potential drug interactions, allergies, and any underlying medical issues are all taken into account when it comes to safety. It is imperative that medical professionals thoroughly evaluate a patient's medical history before recommending or prescribing any herbal therapies or supplements.

In addition, the safety and effectiveness of the vitamins and herbs utilized depend heavily on their quality. Adulterants, contaminants, or subpar goods might reduce or even eliminate the intended health advantages. Therefore, it is essential to purchase herbs and supplements from reliable producers and brands that follow quality assurance guidelines.

CHAPTER EIGHT

MEDICINES AND COMPLEMENTARY THERAPIES

THE FUNCTION OF DRUGS IN FUNCTIONAL MEDICINE

A comprehensive and patient focused approach to treatment, functional medicine aims to treat the underlying causes of disease and enhance general well-being. Even though this paradigm frequently highlights complementary and alternative therapies, pharmaceuticals continue to play a crucial role. Practitioners of functional medicine understand that, when used carefully and in concert with other therapies, drugs can play a significant role in a patient's treatment plan.

In functional medicine, medications are usually used to treat acute or severe illnesses, stabilize the patient's health, or relieve symptoms. For example, medications may be required to treat infections, chronic pain, or specific mental health conditions to manage symptoms and establish a solid foundation for treating underlying issues. In these cases, practitioners of functional medicine explore the role that lifestyle, nutrition, and environment play in the condition while also considering the use of drugs as a stopgap measure.

Furthermore, long-term pharmaceutical management is necessary for certain chronic conditions. Practitioners of functional medicine seek to maximize the use of drugs in these circumstances, frequently by customizing drug selections and dosages to meet the needs of each patient. Additionally, they try to lower the likelihood of side effects and, when feasible, investigate complementary therapies that can lessen the need for pharmaceuticals overall.

INTEGRATING TRADITIONAL AND ALTERNATIVE MEDICINES

The core of functional medicine is integrating the most effective aspects of complementary and alternative therapies to develop a thorough and patient-specific treatment plan. This integration aims to enhance health outcomes by utilizing the advantages of both approaches while acknowledging that each has strengths and limits of its own.

When treating acute diseases and offering prompt relief, conventional procedures like medication and surgery are frequently essential. These procedures are utilized in functional medicine when needed, but they are supplemented by natural therapies such as mind-body practices, acupuncture, chiropractic adjustments, herbal supplements, and dietary changes.

These natural treatments aim to support the body's natural healing processes, deal with the underlying causes of the illness, and enhance general well-being.

In functional medicine, the mix of conventional and natural medicines is customized to meet the specific needs of each patient. It acknowledges that what suits one individual might not be appropriate for another.

Additionally, this method emphasizes preventative care by emphasizing dietary adjustments and lifestyle modifications as ways to lower the risk of chronic illnesses and enhance long-term health.

HANDLING SIDE EFFECTS OF MEDICATION

Adverse drug reactions are a prevalent issue in both conventional and functional medicine. Although many disorders can be effectively treated with medications, side effects are frequently an unexpected consequence of using them. Taking care of these side effects is an essential part of the patient's treatment in functional medicine.

Practitioners of functional medicine evaluate each patient's unique reaction to the medications and try to reduce side effects as much as possible using a variety of strategies. To combat the side effects, this can entail modifying the medicine, upping the dosage, or introducing complementary therapies.

Furthermore, functional medicine's holistic approach enables an emphasis on general health and wellness, which may lessen the need for some prescription drugs. For instance, the patient's health may improve and their dependency on medications may be reduced with lifestyle adjustments such as better nutrition, exercise, stress reduction, and sleep hygiene.

Functional medicine emphasizes the need for a well-rounded strategy that incorporates conventional and complementary therapies to address the underlying causes of illnesses, while also acknowledging the usefulness of pharmaceuticals in specific circumstances.

A key component of this strategy is the control of drug side effects, with an emphasis on reducing their effects and looking into alternate ways to preserve health and well-being.

CHAPTER NINE

DETOXING AND ENVIRONMENTAL HEALTH

METHODS FOR DETOXIFICATION

An essential part of the body's natural defense system against pollutants and dangerous substances in the environment is detoxification. Toxins and waste products must be eliminated to preserve general health and well-being. The body's detoxification processes can be supported and improved by a variety of methods and techniques.

A key component of detoxification is a healthy diet. Eating a diet high in vitamins, minerals, and antioxidants can aid the body's detoxification and neutralization of pollutants. Whole grains, fruits, and vegetables are renowned for their ability to cleanse the body. In addition, it's critical to sustain the body's natural detoxification processes by drinking enough water and herbal teas.

Liver health is another essential component of detoxification. The main organ in charge of breaking down and detoxifying dangerous substances is the liver. Effective toxin removal can be facilitated by maintaining a healthy diet and lifestyle that supports liver function and reducing alcohol and caffeine usage. Several herbal medicines and therapies are said to support liver function, such as dandelion root and milk thistle.

The body naturally gets rid of pollutants through sweating. Regular exercise, saunas, and hot baths can help stimulate the skin's ability to expel pollutants. Exercise increases circulation, which facilitates the effective removal of waste products, in addition to encouraging perspiration.

Additionally, certain procedures and treatments like chelation therapy, intravenous nutrition infusions, and colon cleansing may be part of the detoxification process. In therapeutic settings, these techniques are frequently employed to treat toxin excess or particular medical disorders. However, before pursuing any of these treatments, it's imperative to speak with a licensed healthcare provider.

HEALTH AND ENVIRONMENTAL TOXINS

Toxins found in the environment can come from a variety of sources, such as chemicals, pollution, industrial processes, and even natural sources. The health of humans can be significantly impacted by exposure to these poisons. Certain environmental pollutants, like pesticides, heavy metals, air and water pollutants, and endocrine-disrupting substances, are well-established, whereas the possible health effects of other pollutants are still being investigated.

For example, air pollution is a common environmental toxin that can cause neurological diseases, cardiovascular problems, and respiratory problems. Common causes of contaminated air include particulate matter, volatile chemical compounds, and heavy metals like lead and mercury.

Contamination of water is yet another serious issue. When ingested or utilized in regular activities, contaminants such as lead, arsenic, and chlorine byproducts can find their way into the water supply and constitute a health risk. Neurological and developmental disorders are among the many health concerns that can arise from prolonged exposure to these drugs.

The effects of endocrine-disrupting chemicals (EDCs) on human health have drawn more attention in recent years. EDCs, which include phthalates and bisphenol A (BPA), can disrupt the endocrine system, causing hormonal imbalances and perhaps exacerbating diseases like cancer, obesity, and reproductive issues.

ESTABLISHING A SALUBRIOUS HOME

To reduce exposure to environmental pollutants and promote general well-being, it is imperative to create a healthy living environment. This entails making deliberate decisions in several facets of daily living to lower the toxic load and foster a healthy home environment.

Reducing indoor air pollution is a critical first step in creating a healthy living environment. This can be accomplished by employing air purifiers, appropriately ventilating dwelling areas, and reducing the usage of artificial scents and hazardous cleaning supplies. Maintaining clean indoor air can also be facilitated by selecting furnishings and paints with low volatile organic compounds (VOCs).

Reducing exposure to dangerous chemicals found in personal care items is yet another crucial component of a healthy home. Chemicals found in many skincare products and cosmetics can be absorbed via the skin. Choosing natural and organic products can help promote healthier skin and lower exposure to toxins because they are devoid of toxic substances like phthalates and parabens.

Encouraging personal and environmental health can result from implementing sustainable and eco-friendly activities in the home. Reducing trash, recycling, using water-efficient appliances, and recycling are a few sustainable practices that help

Detoxification techniques are essential for preserving health because they aid the body's natural process of getting rid of pollutants. It is equally vital to understand environmental contaminants and how they affect health since they empower people to make educated decisions and establish healthy living environments. People can take proactive measures to protect their health and lower their exposure to environmental pollutants by adopting these ideas into their daily lives.

CHAPTER TEN

USING FUNCTIONAL MEDICINE TO AGE WELL

SENIOR HEALTH AND LIFESPAN

With the world's population continuing to age, the notions of geriatric health and longevity are closely related and have received more attention recently. Geriatrics is the study of the healthcare requirements of elderly people to improve their longevity and quality of life. The objective of aging gracefully is complex and includes mental and emotional as well as physical wellness. In this effort, functional medicine is essential because it addresses the underlying causes of age-related health problems and promotes patient-centered, comprehensive care.

When it comes to aging gracefully, longevity means not just living a longer life but also living a longer life with vigor and good health. Although our longevity is largely determined by our genes, a variety of circumstances, such as lifestyle decisions, dietary habits, and medical procedures, all have an impact on how we age and the quality of our later years. Functional medicine seeks to increase not only the quantity but also the quality of years lived by acknowledging the significance of individualized and preventive care. It recognizes that every person's aging process is unique and that there is no one-size-fits-all solution.

STANDARD AGE-RELATED HEALTH CONCERNS

While age-related health problems are an inherent aspect of growing older, we do not have to accept this as the end of the road. To address these problems, functional medicine first determines their underlying causes before creating plans to control and lessen their effects. The following are a few typical age-related health problems:

1. Cardiovascular Health: Heart disease, high blood pressure, and other cardiovascular problems become more likely as people age. A key component of functional medicine is the management of heart health by dietary, physical activity, and stress reduction changes in lifestyle.

2. Cognitive Decline: With diseases like dementia and Alzheimer's disease becoming more common, cognitive decline is a major issue for older persons. To address cognitive health, functional medicine focuses on diets that improve brain function, lifestyle modifications, and the identification and treatment of possible causes for cognitive decline.

3. Osteoporosis: As people age, they often experience a reduction in bone density, which increases their risk of fractures. To preserve bone health, functional medicine suggests consuming foods that build bones and engaging in weight-bearing activities.

4. Hormonal Changes: As people become older, hormonal imbalances are increasingly common and can cause a variety of symptoms like mood swings, hot flashes, and decreased libido. To properly manage these changes, functional medicine provides individualized treatments through hormone replacement medication and lifestyle modifications.

5. Digestive Health: Age-related digestive problems can exacerbate and impair nutrient absorption as well as general health. To improve digestion, functional medicine practitioners emphasize gut health, diet change, and identifying food sensitivities.

6. Musculoskeletal Issues: Two typical concerns among older persons are musculoskeletal discomfort and arthritis. Functional medicine uses complementary and alternative methods, such as food, physical therapy, and supplements, to treat pain and inflammation.

7. Metabolic Syndrome: Changes in metabolism brought on by aging may result in insulin resistance, weight gain, and other metabolic problems. Personalized diet plans and lifestyle modifications are used in functional medicine to promote metabolic health and ward off related diseases like diabetes.

Longevity and geriatric health are related, and functional medicine is essential to promoting healthy aging. Functional medicine looks for the underlying causes of common age-related health problems and emphasizes a tailored, holistic approach to therapy to improve overall well-being and quality of life into later life. While acknowledging that aging is a normal part of life, it also holds that people can live longer, healthier, and more satisfying lives if they employ the appropriate techniques and interventions.

www.ingramcontent.com/pod-product-compliance
Lightning Source LLC
Chambersburg PA
CBHW060804260726
48660CB00002B/765